L-THEANINE

Enhance Focus, Reduce Stress, and Achieve Mental Clarity with Nature's Calming Secret By Unlocking the Power of L-Theanine

SAMANTHA ZYLAR

Contents

CHAPTER ONE

Overview

Finding calm in the hectic, fast-paced world of today can seem like an unattainable goal. Many of us long for a break from the everyday chaos brought on by the pressures of work, the bustle of the city, and the continual presence of digital screens clamoring for our attention.

You're in for a treat if you've ever wondered whether there's a natural approach to de-stress, improve attention, and discover serenity. Introducing L-theanine, a special amino acid with amazing qualities that can assist you in regaining your equilibrium.

The Path To L-Theanine Discovery

L-Theanine, a chemical present in the leaves of the tea plant Camellia sinensis, is where our adventure started. L-Theanine has been consumed for generations in tea-drinking countries such as Japan, China, and Taiwan, but the Western world has only just begun to realize its full potential. Because of its significant effects on the body and mind, it has attracted the attention of scientists, who have conducted several studies and gathered a growing body of information on its various advantages.

We will examine the origins of L-theanine and the cultural traditions that shed light on this amazing amino acid as we delve into its history in this book. We'll also look more closely at how contemporary science has increased and validated our understanding of the potential benefits of L-theanine, making it more accessible to individuals looking for natural remedies for their health issues.

This Particular Amino Acid's Power

You will quickly learn that L-theanine is not your typical amino acid. It possesses the rare capacity to pass through the blood-brain barrier and alter brain chemistry in ways that both encourage alertness and relaxation. L-theanine is a popular natural cure for a variety of problems, from stress and anxiety to enhanced cognitive performance and better sleep quality. Its dual effect sets it apart from other drugs.

We shall examine the many possible advantages of L-theanine as well as the methods by which it has a calming effect on the brain throughout this book. You'll learn about its benefits for managing anxiety and stress, as well as how it might improve your meditation experience. We'll also talk about how L-Theanine works well with other supplements, like caffeine, to give a well-balanced increase of energy and mental clarity without giving users the jitters that come with caffeine use.

Anticipations For This Book

You may anticipate a thorough investigation of L-theanine across this book's pages, including information on its origins, history, and modes of action. We'll talk about its possible uses and how to implement it into your daily schedule to reap the first rewards. This book has something to teach everyone, whether you're a tea fan trying to learn the science behind your favorite beverage or someone searching for a natural solution to boost mental clarity and reduce stress.

We will include helpful hints, suggested dosages, and updates on the most recent L-theanine research across the chapters. By the time you finish reading these pages, you'll have a profound respect for the effectiveness of L-theanine and a fresh awareness of how it may lead to a life that is more peaceful, focused, and healthful.

Knowledge Of L-Theanine

L-theanine is an intriguing amino acid that has been more well-known recently due to its unusual qualities and possible health advantages.

Let's examine L-theanine's function in relation to amino acids, its unique characteristics, and its natural sources in order to have a better understanding of the compound.

A Synopsis Of Amino Acids In Brief:

The building blocks of proteins and amino acids are essential to many physiological functions carried out by the human body. The creation of proteins, enzymes, neurotransmitters, and other critical components depends on these chemical substances.

Three categories are commonly used to categorize amino acids: essential, non-essential, and conditional. The body is unable to produce essential amino acids, so it must get them from food.

Among the amino acids that are not necessary is L-theanine. The body can manufacture non-essential amino acids, but it can also obtain them through diet. Unlike most other amino acids, leucine is not utilized in the creation of proteins, making it a unique amino acid. Rather, it affects the body and brain in a variety of distinctive ways.

What Is Unique About L-Theanine?

1. Relaxation and Stress Reduction: One of L-Theanine's most remarkable properties is its capacity to encourage relaxation without making one feel

sleepy. It accomplishes this by boosting the generation of alpha brain waves, which are linked to a relaxed, awake state. For this reason, L-Theanine is frequently used in supplements meant to lower anxiety and stress levels.

2. L-theanine is frequently taken in conjunction with caffeine because it might lessen the jittery and anxious adverse effects of caffeine intake. It enhances focus and alertness without the anxiety that goes along with caffeine's stimulating effects.

3. L-theanine has been demonstrated to improve cognitive performance. It can enhance learning, memory, and

concentration, which makes it a desirable choice for people looking for nootropic advantages.

4. L-theanine has been demonstrated in certain trials to enhance the quality of sleep by facilitating relaxation and shortening the time it takes to fall asleep. This makes it a fascinating supplement for people who have problems sleeping.

Natural L-Theanine Sources:

The most frequent source of L-theanine is tea leaves, namely those of the Camellia sinensis plant, which produces black, green, and white tea.

various tea varieties have various concentrations of L-theanine, with green tea often having higher levels than black tea. To extract L-Theanine from tea, one merely needs to steep the leaves in hot water and then consume the beverage.

Aside from tea, L-Theanine can also be found in smaller concentrations in certain edible mushrooms, such as Xerocomus badius, and some kinds of seaweed. But tea is still the most accessible and well-liked natural source of L-theanine.

In summary, L-theanine is a special kind of non-essential amino acid that may have a number of positive effects on health, especially in the areas of stress relief, relaxation, improved sleep, and cognitive function. Because of its natural sources, which are mostly found in tea, those who want to use it to improve their well-being can simply acquire it.

The Science Behind L-Theanine

An amino acid called L-theanine is found naturally in tea leaves, especially in green tea (Camellia sinensis). Its possible advantages for improving mood, lowering stress levels, and cognitive performance have drawn a lot of interest. It is crucial to investigate L-theanine's effects on the brain, its interactions with neurotransmitters, and the scientific and clinical evidence that backs these claims in order to comprehend the science behind the supplement.

How The Brain Processes L-Theanine:

1. L-theanine is well-known for its capacity to pass through the blood-brain barrier, a semipermeable membrane that divides the brain from the bloodstream. It can therefore directly affect how the brain functions.

2.   Gamma-aminobutyric   acid (GABA) and glutamate are the two main neurotransmitters that L-theanine modifies in order to affect brain function. While glutamate is an excitatory neurotransmitter that is involved in alertness and cognition, GABA   is   an   inhibitory neurotransmitter that encourages relaxation and lowers anxiety.

3. Alpha Brain Waves: It has been noted that L-theanine stimulates the generation of alpha brain waves. These brain waves are frequently observed during profound relaxation and meditation, and they are linked to a state of relaxed alertness. L-theanine may have a soothing and focalizing

effect because it increases alpha waves.

The Interaction Of L-Theanine With Neurotransmitters:

1. GABAergic Effects: L-theanine has the ability to raise brain GABA levels. This rise in GABA activity has the potential to lessen tension and anxiety while fostering a calmer state of mind.

2. Effects on Glutamate: L-theanine possesses a special property that prevents glutamate from attaching to its receptors, hence lowering glutamate excitatory activity. This regulation may result in less

overstimulation, better cognitive function, and increased attention.

3. Dopaminergic Effects: Research indicates that L-theanine may have an indirect effect on dopamine release, which is a neurotransmitter linked to motivation and reward. Focus and mood may both improve as a result of this.

Investigations And Clinical Research:

The effects of L-theanine on human health and cognitive function have been the subject of several scientific investigations and clinical trials. Among the important conclusions are:

1. Stress Reduction: Research on both humans and animals has demonstrated that L-theanine lowers stress and anxiety levels. It can promote relaxation without making you drowsy and counteract the stimulating effects of caffeine.

2. Increased Focus and Attention: Studies indicate that combining L-theanine with caffeine may improve focus and cognitive function. It is thought that the mixture provides a harmony between tranquility and attentiveness.

3. Mood Enhancement: Although more research is required in this area, L-theanine has been linked to

enhanced mood and may play a role in controlling symptoms of depression and mood disorders.

4. Sleep Quality: Research suggests that L-theanine may help those who suffer from sleep disorders and enhance the quality of their sleep.

In conclusion, research on L-theanine indicates that it may have a calming, stress-relieving, and cognitively enhancing effect by acting on brain neurotransmitters, specifically glutamate and GABA. Clinical investigations and research back up its potential as a natural substance to enhance mental health and general cognitive function. But before adding

L-Theanine to your daily regimen, like with any supplement or substance, make sure to speak with a healthcare provider. This is especially important if you have any particular health problems or are on medication.

CHAPTER TWO

Advantages Of L-Theanine For Health

Often present in tea leaves, especially in green tea, L-theanine is an amino acid with a number of health advantages. We'll look at its effects on a few important facets of health and well-being here:

1. Reduction Of Tension And Anxiety:

L-theanine is known to help induce relaxation and lower levels of tension and anxiety. Gamma-aminobutyric acid (GABA), a neurotransmitter with relaxing properties in the brain, is produced more when it is used. Because of this, L-theanine is a well-liked natural solution for people looking for a non-pharmacological way to reduce stress and anxiety.

2. Focus And Cognitive Enhancement: L-theanine and caffeine work synergetically to improve cognitive performance. This combination is frequently used. Together, these ingredients can enhance focus, recall, and general cognitive function without causing the jitters or crashes that come with excessive caffeine consumption. It's especially useful for tasks requiring

prolonged focus because it fosters a calm alertness.

3. Improved Sleep Quality:

L-theanine has been associated with improved sleep quality. It can facilitate easier falling asleep and deeper, more restful sleep by encouraging relaxation and lowering stress levels. L-theanine is a natural substitute for sleep aids because of its soothing effects, which also help to reduce the symptoms of insomnia.

4. Potential In Supporting

Cardiovascular Health:

L-theanine has demonstrated potential in supporting cardiovascular health. It can relax blood arteries, which improves blood flow and lowers blood pressure. These benefits have the potential to lower the risk of heart-related disorders and promote heart health.

5. Immune Support:

According to certain research, L-theanine may have the ability to strengthen the immune system. L-theanine is thought to help the immune system by lowering stress and encouraging a balanced, less inflammatory response in the body, though further research in this area is required.

6. Weight Control:

L-theanine's ability to reduce stress and anxiety may help with weight control inadvertently. Stress frequently acts as a catalyst for binge eating and unhealthy food choices. L-theanine may aid with weight loss and maintenance by lowering stress and emotional eating.

Although L-theanine is usually regarded as safe and well-tolerated, individual reactions may differ. See a healthcare provider before incorporating it into your regular routine or using it as a supplement, particularly if you are taking medication or have any underlying medical conditions. Including L-theanine in a healthy, balanced diet may have a major positive impact on many areas of your health and well-being.

L-Theanine And Emotional Wellbeing

An amino acid called L-theanine is present naturally in tea leaves, especially in green tea. Its potential to support mental health and well-being has drawn attention. The relationship between L-theanine and mental health is explored in this idea, which includes how it affects depression, anxiety disorders, and stress management while enhancing mental health in general.

1. L-Theanine And Anxiety Disorders:

Millions of people worldwide suffer from anxiety disorders, which are among the most prevalent mental health issues. L-theanine has demonstrated the potential to reduce the symptoms associated with anxiety. It is well known that this amino acid helps people unwind without making them feel sleepy. It funct ions by raising the concentrations of neurotransmitters linked to calmness, such as serotonin and GABA (gamma-aminobutyric acid). L-theanine may lessen anxiety symptoms such as excessive worrying, restlessness, and uneasiness by regulating these neurotransmitters.

Many people discover that drinking green tea or taking L-theanine supplements can have a relaxing effect and aid in the management of anxiety.

2. L-Theanine In Depression:

Depression is a mood-altering, multifaceted mental

health illness that frequently leaves sufferers with enduring depressive and gloomy sentiments. Due to its capacity to increase serotonin and other neurotransmitter activities, L-theanine may play a part in depression.

Depression and low serotonin levels are frequently linked. Because of its relaxing qualities and effect on serotonin, L-theanine may help lessen the symptoms of depression. Although it is not a cure-all for depression, when combined with other therapeutic methods, it may prove to be a useful adjunctive strategy.

3. Fighting Stress And Encouraging Mental

Health: Chronic stress can result in a number of mental health issues. Stress is a common concern in our fast-paced, contemporary life. The ability of L-theanine to reduce stress has drawn attention. It can lessen the negative effects of stress on the body and mind, including elevated heart rate and anxiety. L-theanine supports general mental health by encouraging relaxation and lowering stress perception. Many people discover that drinking tea or supplements containing L-theanine improves their ability to relax and cope with stress.

It's crucial to remember that even though L-theanine may have positive effects on mental health, it shouldn't take the place of professional mental health care when needed. For an appropriate diagnosis and course of treatment, those experiencing severe anxiety disorders, depression, or other mental health concerns should speak with healthcare professionals.

To sum up, research on the effects of L-theanine on mental health is intriguing and shows promise in enhancing mental health, reducing anxiety, and possibly even helping to manage depression.

Adding L-Theanine to one's diet—via supplements or dietary sources like green tea—may provide a beneficial adjunctive strategy for promoting mental health and emotional stability in general. Before making any major adjustments to one's mental health treatment plan, it is advisable to speak with a healthcare expert because individual reactions may differ.

L-Theanine And Mental Abilities

Natural amino acid L-theanine is mostly present in tea leaves, especially in green tea, and is well known for its possible ability to improve cognitive function. L-theanine has drawn attention for its beneficial effects on three major areas of cognitive function: improving focus and concentration, improving memory, and increasing creativity.

1. Increasing Focus And Concentration:

L-theanine is frequently commended for its capacity to encourage a calm, aware state of mind. It accomplishes this by boosting the synthesis of neurotransmitters that aid in mood and attention regulation, such as serotonin and dopamine. L-theanine can increase concentration and attention span without having the jittery side effects that are sometimes connected to stimulants like caffeine since it fosters a calm, concentrated state of mind.

Research has indicated that L-theanine can improve attention and concentration when combined with caffeine, a common stimulant. L-theanine plus caffeine is thought to retain caffeine's stimulating benefits on cognitive performance while reducing its negative side effects, such as anxiety and restlessness.

2. Memory

Augmentation: Another area where L-theanine has demonstrated potential is memory augmentation. The relaxing properties of L-theanine have been proposed to help lessen stress and anxiety, two conditions known to impede memory. L-theanine may improve working memory and cognitive processing by inducing a relaxed mood. Additionally, some research has indicated that L-theanine may have a neuroprotective impact, which may be advantageous for maintaining long-term brain health.

L-theanine may help reduce stress in addition to raising levels of brain-derived neurotrophic factor (BDNF), a protein linked to cognitive function and memory formation. This could provide even more insight into L-theanine's ability to improve memory.

3. Enhancing Creativity:

Being open-minded and at ease can help foster creativity, which is a sophisticated cognitive process. The capacity of L-theanine to induce relaxation without inducing sleepiness can be utilized to enhance creativity. L-theanine may assist people in overcoming mental obstacles and inhibitions that impede creative thought by lowering tension and anxiety.

L-theanine's interaction with neurotransmitters such as dopamine and serotonin can also help elevate mood, which is frequently associated with higher levels of creativity.

In conclusion, research has linked L-theanine to a number of cognitive advantages, such as improved focus and attention, improved memory, and increased creativity. It is a supplement that appeals to people who want to maximize cognitive function without experiencing the negative effects of conventional stimulants because of its special ability to promote relaxation and mood regulation. L-theanine is a promising natural supplement for those wishing to boost their cognitive well-being, while individual reactions may differ.

CHAPTER THREE

L-Theanine And Well-Being

L-Theanine is an amino acid largely present in tea leaves, notably in green tea, and is known for its possible favorable benefits on physical health. While it is widely appreciated for its role in encouraging relaxation and lowering stress, L-Theanine may also offer various benefits relating to physical well-being. Here, we'll study how L-Theanine may help areas of physical health, including decreasing blood pressure, immune system support, weight management, and skin health.

1. Lowering Blood Pressure:

Pressure: L-Theanine has been associated with promoting relaxation and reducing anxiety, partly by increasing the production of calming neurotransmitters like GABA (gamma-aminobutyric acid) in the brain. This relaxation response may extend to the cardiovascular system, where L-Theanine has shown potential in reducing blood pressure. L-theanine is sometimes taken with coffee to help counterbalance its stimulating effects, according to studies. This combination is well-liked by people who want to keep their blood pressure in check without compromising attentiveness.

2. Immune System Support: L-Theanine has proven immune-enhancing qualities in various research. It may promote the formation of certain immune cells, including T cells and natural killer cells, which play key roles in the body's defense against infections and disorders. L-theanine may improve general physical health by strengthening the immune system and enabling the body to fight off infections more successfully.

3. Weight Management:

Weight management is closely linked to physical health, and L-Theanine may indirectly support healthy weight management. The relaxation and stress-reduction effects of L-Theanine can help reduce stress-related overeating and emotional eating, which are common contributors to weight gain. L-Theanine may also help people stick to their workout and weight loss plans by improving focus and concentration.

4. Skin Health: Although the

connection between L-Theanine and skin health is less explored than other aspects of its benefits, some researchers have suggested that the amino acid's antioxidant properties could have a positive impact. Antioxidants aid in shielding the skin from oxidative stress, which can hasten the aging process and result in a number of skin disorders. The possible stress-reduction benefits of L-theanine may potentially tangentially improve skin health by easing stress-related skin conditions including eczema and acne.

It's crucial to remember that although L-theanine may have certain advantages, each person may have different impacts from it. Integrating L-Theanine into a healthy, balanced lifestyle that includes regular exercise, a well-rounded diet, and other stress-reduction methods may be the best way to fully reap these advantages. It is essential to speak with a healthcare provider before taking L-theanine supplements for specific health goals to make sure they are in line with personal needs, current medications, and any existing ailments.

Including L-Theanine In Your Everyday Diet

An amino acid called L-theanine is naturally present in tea leaves, especially in green tea, and is well-known for its ability to promote calmness and relaxation. Adding L-

Theanine to your daily regimen can be beneficial, particularly if you want to lower stress, sharpen your focus, or get better sleep. This is how you do it:

1. Guidelines For Safety And Dosage:

• Dosage: 200–400 mg per day is the usual dosage for L-theanine supplements. For improved cognitive function, it's frequently used with caffeine.

• Safety: It is generally accepted that L-theanine is safe and well-tolerated. Addiction or drowsiness are not caused by it. To gauge your individual response, it's best to begin with a lesser dosage and progressively raise it as necessary.

2. Selecting Appropriate Supplements:

• Purity and Quality: Choose reliable brands and look for L-theanine supplements that have undergone independent testing to ensure both purity and quality.

• Capsules or Powder: There are two different kinds of L-theanine: capsules and powder. Which of the two you choose will rely on your personal preferences. While powder can be added to drinks, capsules are more handy and straightforward to dose.

3. Timing:

• Morning: Consider taking L-Theanine in the morning with your breakfast or alongside your morning coffee for a more focused and alert start to the day.

• Evening: L-Theanine can also be taken in the evening to help with relaxation and sleep. It's a great option if you have difficulty falling asleep.

4. Combining Tea With L-Theanine:

• Green Tea: Include green tea in your routine if you'd rather get your L-Theanine naturally. Green tea powder, or matcha, has a high content of L-Theanine.

• Tea Breaks: To reduce stress and preserve mental clarity, take brief L-Theanine breaks throughout the day by sipping a cup of tea.

5. Continuity:

• Consistency is crucial when introducing L-Theanine into your everyday routine. Regular use can lead to more obvious and prolonged benefits, especially in relation to stress reduction and enhanced attention.

6. Monitoring Effects:

• Pay attention to how L-Theanine affects you. Some people could report a more rapid soothing effect, while others may notice better focus and cognitive performance. Adjust your dosage or time based on your particular needs.

L-Theanine In Combination With Other Supplements:

L-theanine can be taken in combination with other supplements to maximize its benefits or target particular health objectives. Consider the following combinations:

1. Coffee With L-Theanine:

• L-theanine and caffeine together are well-liked for their synergistic effects. L-theanine can increase alertness and focus by reducing the jittery or nervous feeling that coffee can cause.

2. Galectin With L-Theanine:

• Gamma-aminobutyric acid, GABA, and L-theanine together can promote calmness and lessen anxiety. Another neurotransmitter that helps induce serenity is GABA, and when combined, the two can have an even more noticeable relaxing impact.

3. Melatonin With L-Theanine:

• Melatonin and L-theanine together may help enhance the quality of your sleep. Melatonin controls your sleep-wake cycle, whereas L-theanine aids in relaxation.

4. L-Theanine With Adaptogens From Herbs:

• Combining L-Theanine with herbal adaptogens such as rhodiola or ashwagandha can offer a comprehensive strategy for reducing stress and enhancing general health.

Recall that you should always speak with a healthcare provider before taking L-Theanine in combination with other supplements, particularly if you have any underlying medical conditions or are on medication. They can assist in making sure the combinations are suitable and safe for your unique requirements.

CHAPTER FOUR
Useful Instances And Recipes

Natural amino acids like L-theanine are frequently found in tea leaves, especially in green tea. It is renowned for its exceptional capacity to promote serenity and relaxation while preserving mental clarity. Due to its usefulness in many facets of daily life, this compound has garnered attention. We will go over the useful uses of L-theanine in this conversation and offer some recipes to assist you in incorporating it into your daily routine.

Making The Optimal L-Theanine-Rich Tea

A quick and easy method to feel the relaxing effects of L-Theanine is to brew a cup of tea that's high in the amino acid. The following advice will help you make the ideal cup:

1. Select the Right Tea: If you're looking to drink tea, go for green tea. High-quality loose-leaf kinds are especially good because they have a higher L-Theanine content than black or oolong teas.

2. Fresh tea leaves are best because quality matters. Think about spending money on premium tea because they

frequently have a stronger L-Theanine concentration.

3. Water Temperature: Use water heated to roughly 175°F (80°C) for green tea. Bitterness is avoided by the sensitive L-Theanine components being preserved at this lower temperature.

4. Steep With Mindfulness: The recommended amount of time to steep green tea is one to two minutes, though this can vary. To suit your tastes, adjust as necessary, but don't overstep as this could result in an unpleasant aftertaste.

5. Savor Calmly: To maximize the relaxing effects of L-Theanine, make

your tea-drinking experience as peaceful as possible. The calming effects of the amino acid can be enhanced with a brief period of mindfulness.

Recipes With L-Theanine Infusion

There are many inventive ways to include L-Theanine in your everyday diet besides making tea. Here are some ideas for recipes:

1.   Smoothie with L-theanine Infusion:

• Combine Greek yogurt, honey, green tea leaves, and fresh fruit (such as bananas or mangos). The addition of green tea leaves to the smoothie will provide both an earthy flavor and L-Theanine.

2. Salads Enhanced with L-Theanine:

Mix matcha, or powdered green tea, into your vinaigrette. Matcha's mild bitterness works well with lemon, honey, and olive oil to create a special salad dressing.

3. Latte with Theanine:

• Combine matcha with a little honey, warm milk, and cinnamon. This warming drink provides a pleasant L-Theanine hit.

4. Desserts Infused with L-Theanine:

Try experimenting with your dessert recipes by adding matcha or green tea. Delightful options include matcha-infused chocolates, green tea ice cream, and matcha cookies.

Using L-Theanine In Everyday Life

L-theanine may enter your daily routine in a number of ways, including:

1. Tension Relief: To assist in lowering tension and anxiety levels, take a break from your busy schedule and sip on a cup of tea high in the amino acid L-theanine.

2. Productivity at Work: L-theanine has been reported by some to improve attention and concentration. To keep your mind clear when working or studying, think about drinking tea.

3. Sleep Aid: Including L-theanine in your nighttime regimen may be beneficial. It could be simpler to unwind and go to asleep if you have a cup of decaffeinated green tea before bed.

4. Social and Relaxation: Share a pot of tea with friends and family to establish a peaceful and friendly mood during gatherings.

In conclusion, L-Theanine is a versatile molecule with several practical applications in your daily life. Whether you're seeking relaxation, better productivity, or a unique culinary experience, L-Theanine-rich tea and recipes can be a helpful addition to your routine, bringing both flavor and a sense of serenity.

Conclusion

L-Theanine, a unique amino acid largely found in tea leaves, has attracted substantial interest in recent years for its possible health benefits and cognitive-enhancing characteristics. As we complete our investigation of L-Theanine, it's crucial to emphasize its many advantages and acknowledge its hopeful future in various sectors.

Summarizing The Benefits Of L-Theanine:

L-Theanine offers a wide range of benefits. One of the most well-known advantages is its ability to promote relaxation and reduce stress and anxiety without causing drowsiness. This calming effect is often attributed to its ability to increase the levels of neurotransmitters such as GABA and dopamine in the brain. As a result, L-Theanine has been explored as a natural remedy for stress management and may complement traditional therapies for anxiety disorders.

Additionally, L-Theanine is sometimes used in concert with caffeine to produce a balanced energy increase. It can help mitigate the jitters and crashes that come with taking caffeine, which makes it a useful ingredient in energy pills and nootropic stacks. Its relaxing and focus-enhancing properties make it a popular option for anyone looking to boost their cognitive function.

L-theanine may also have neuroprotective qualities. According to certain research, it might lessen the incidence of age-related neurodegenerative disorders and cognitive loss by shielding brain cells from harm.

Prospective Research And Its Possible Uses:

Future research has intriguing new directions to explore thanks to the potential benefits of L-theanine. Scholars are currently investigating its possible uses in a number of domains, such as:

1. Mental Health: More investigation into the effectiveness and safety of L-theanine as an adjuvant treatment for anxiety and stress-related illnesses may yield important new information.

2.	Cognitive	Enhancement:
Researching L-Theanine's long-term effects on memory and cognitive function may have significant ramifications for people looking to sharpen their focus and focus.

3. Neuroprotection: Further research into the possible neuroprotective qualities of L-theanine may lead to the development of novel treatments for neurodegenerative illnesses including Parkinson's and Alzheimer's.

4. Enhancement of Sleep: Due to its soothing properties, L-theanine is used in supplements and sleep aids. Further investigation may assist in

maximizing its application in encouraging sound sleep.

The Way Ahead:

It is important that we proceed with caution and enthusiasm when discussing L-theanine. More thorough clinical trials are required to validate and improve our comprehension of this amino acid's potential uses, even though the volume of data that is already available points to a number of possible advantages.

It is important for customers to understand the potency and quality of L-theanine supplements as well as any possible interactions with other drugs or medical issues. To ensure safe and efficient use, speaking with medical specialists and adhering to authorized dosages are crucial.

To sum up, research on L-theanine is intriguing and has the potential to improve mental health, cognitive performance, and general well-being. It is an all-natural, secure, and easily-acquired instrument that has already proven useful in a number of situations.

We might be able to confirm its place in the fields of healthcare and wellness and unearth even more of its untapped potential with continued investigation.

9 798870 169026